THIS BOOK BELONGS TO:

_____

Some suggestions on how to use this book:

This journal can be used to explore your thoughts and feelings about your hair in the form of writing and drawing. Feel free to use it in a way that makes the most sense to you. You may find that you only want to write out your thoughts or you may feel that some things are better expressed with a drawing or both! There are also some pages in the back that don't have any prompts for you to answer. You can use those to express new thoughts you may have about your hair The most important thing is to know that this book will help you learn more about your hair and how your hair makes you feel.

My hair looks like

Do you like the way your hair looks?

My hair feels like

Do you like the way your hair feels?

My hair smells like

Do you like the way your hair smells?

My hair color is

Do you like your hair color?

My hair length is

Do you like your hair length?

My hair is washed every

My hair is deep conditioned every

Wash day makes me feel

My scalp is greased every

When my mama greases my scalp, it feels

When my mama combs my hair, it feels

When my mama brushes my hair, it feels

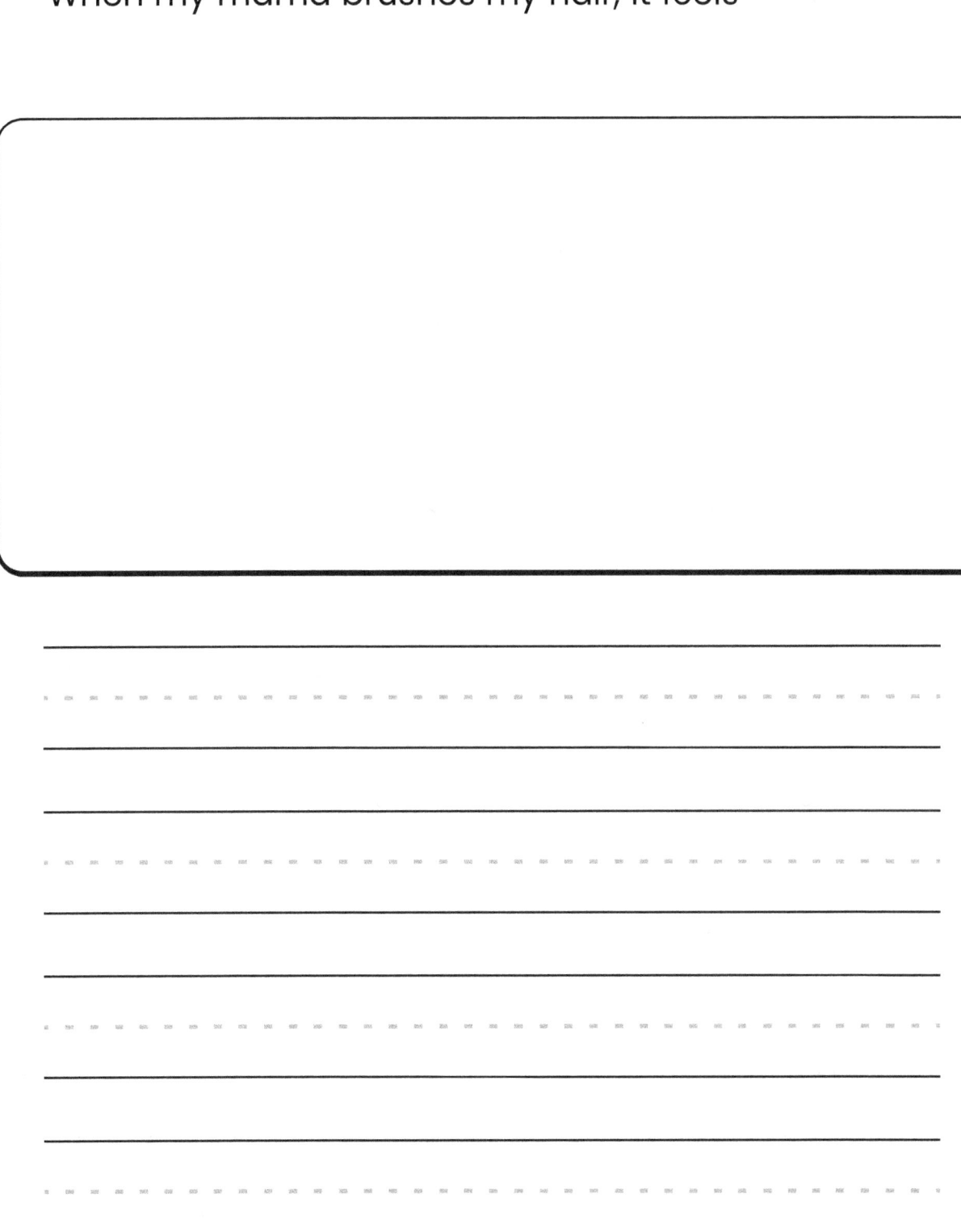

Three words that describe my hair are

My favorite hairstyle is

My least favorite hairstyle is

Before I go to bed, I do this to my hair

In the morning, I do this to my hair

My favorite type of braids is

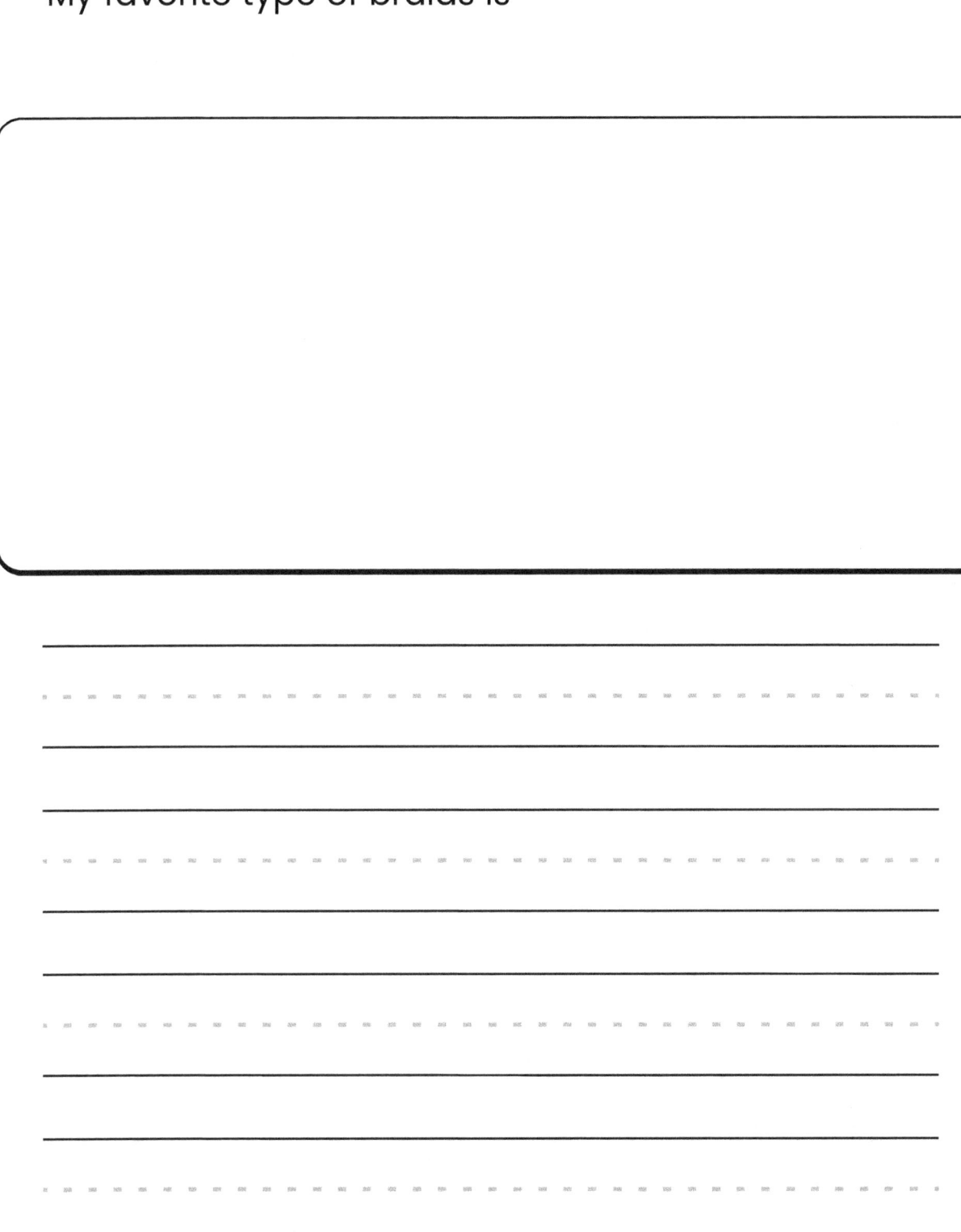

My favorite type of ponytail is

Wearing my hair down feels

A new, fresh hairstyle makes me feel

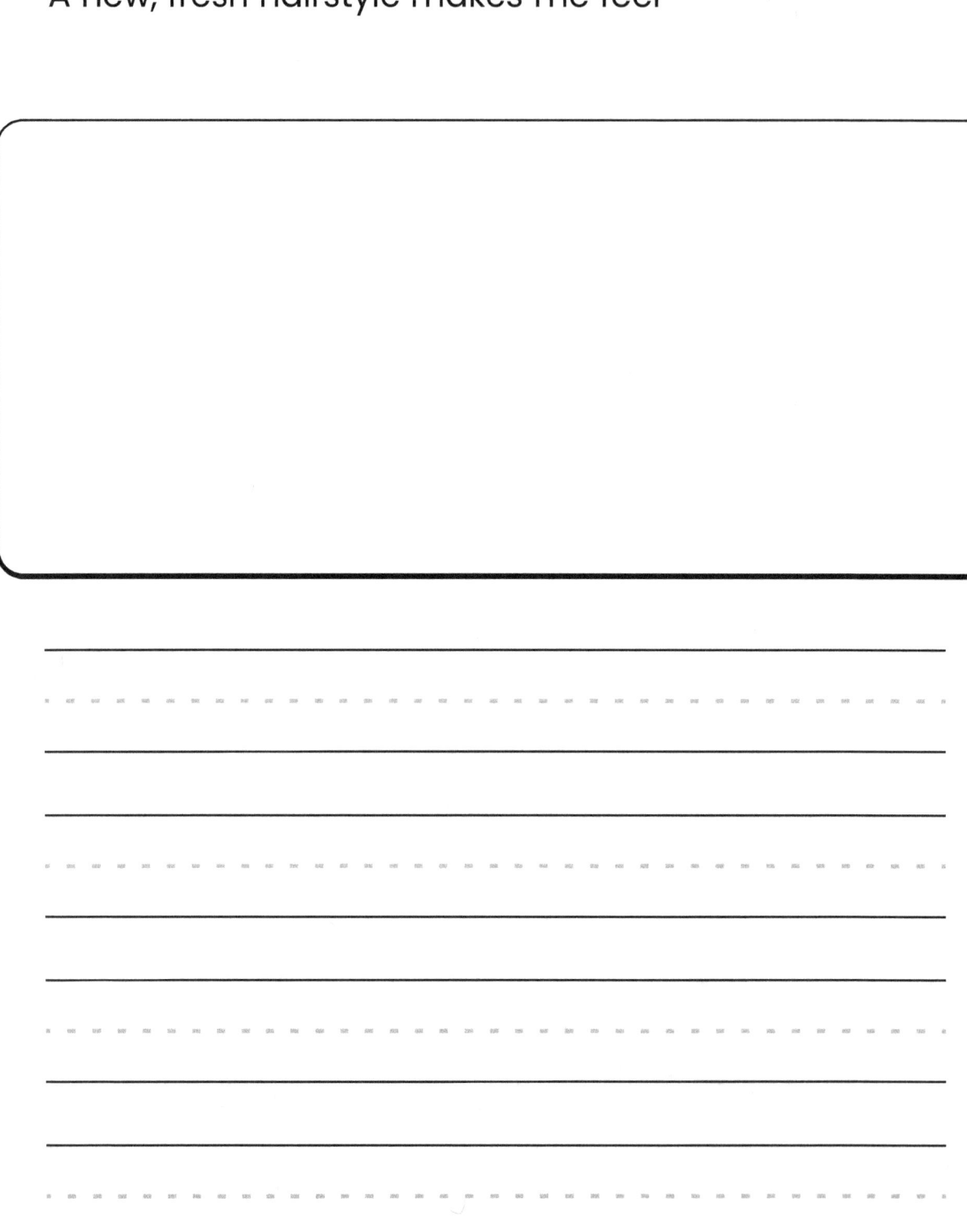

An old hairstyle makes me feel

I like my hair because

I don't like my hair because

I wish my hair was more

I wish my hair was less

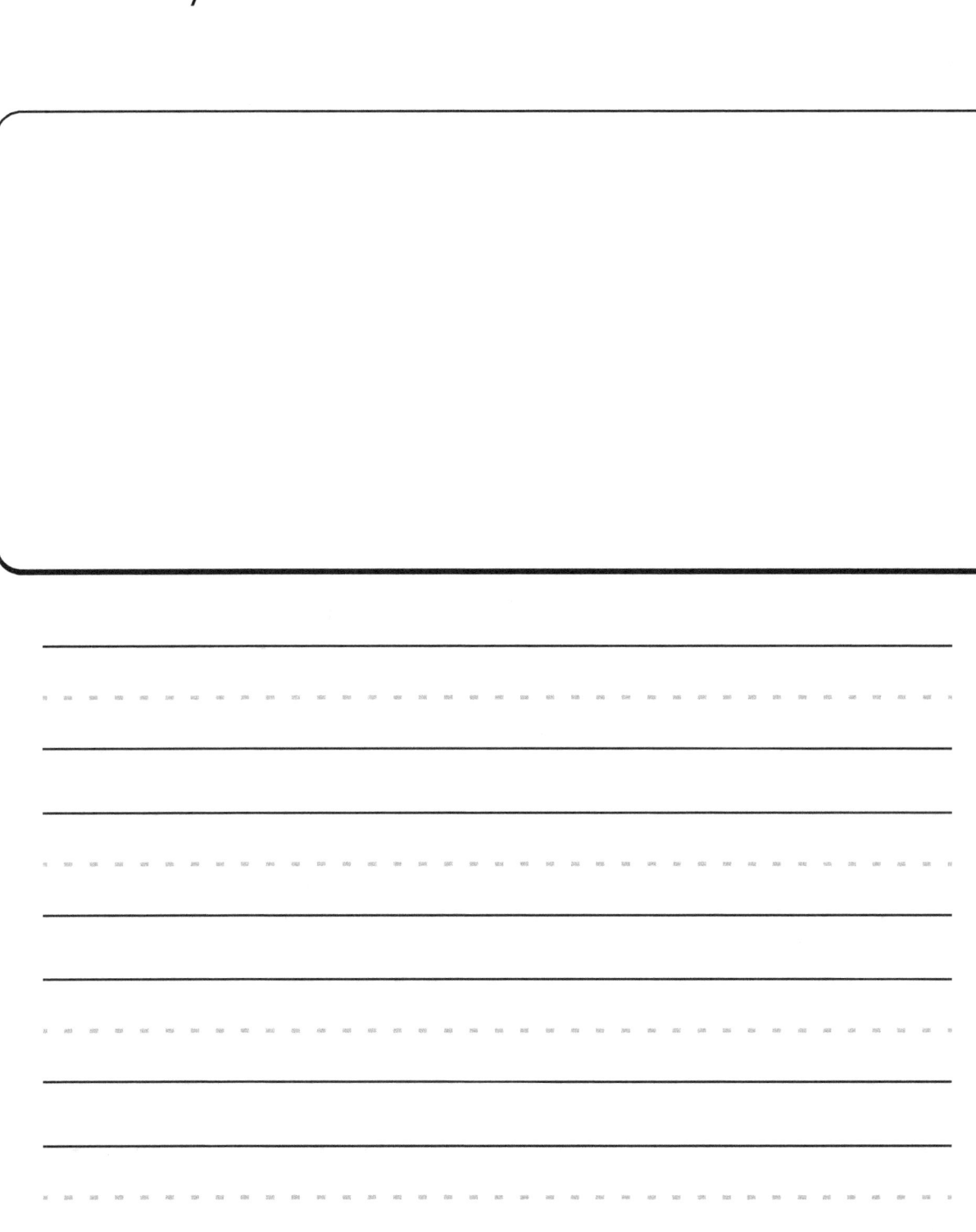

If I could change my hair color, it would be

If I could change my hair length, it would be

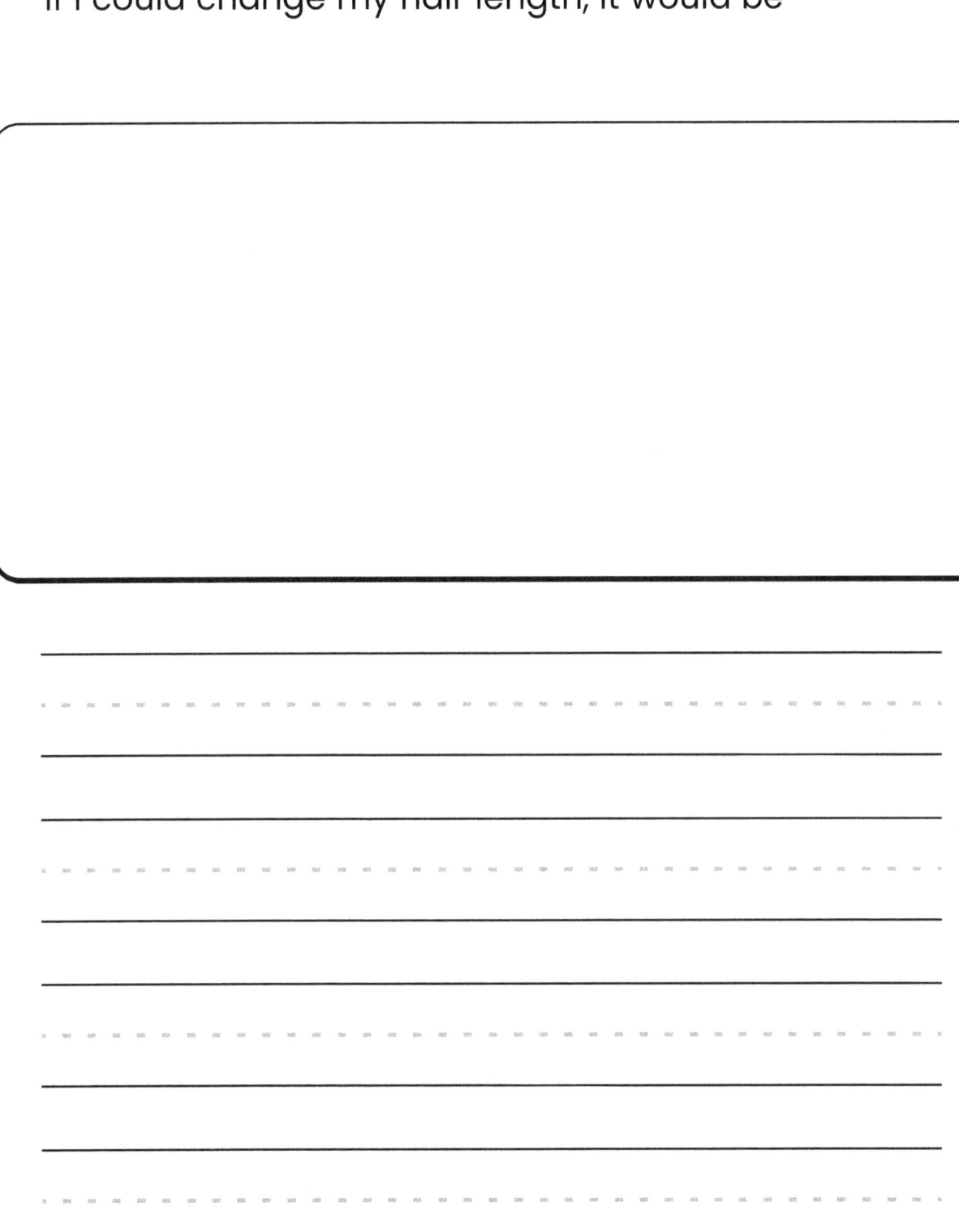

If I could change my hair texture, it would be

Kids at school have said that my hair is

I think long hair is

I think straight hair is

I think an afro is

I think an afro feels like

_____

_____

_____

_____

_____

_____

Asking to touch my hair is

Touching my hair without asking is

My favorite color to wear in my hair is

Some things I like to wear in my hair are

I like barrettes in the shape of

I like beads that look like

When I grow up, I will wear my hair like

My mama's hair as a girl looked like

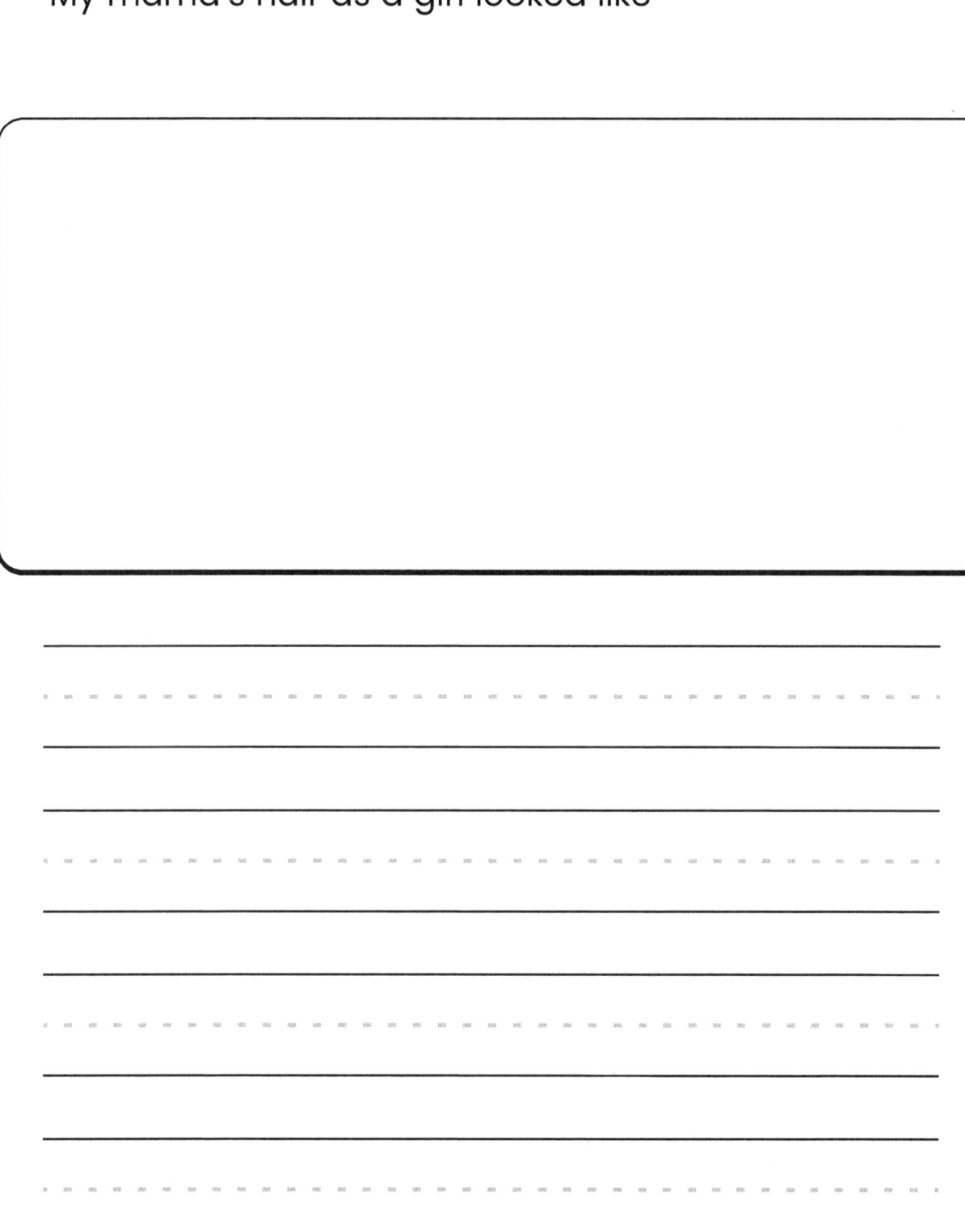

My mama's hair looks like

Combing my mama's hair would be

My mama thinks that her hair is

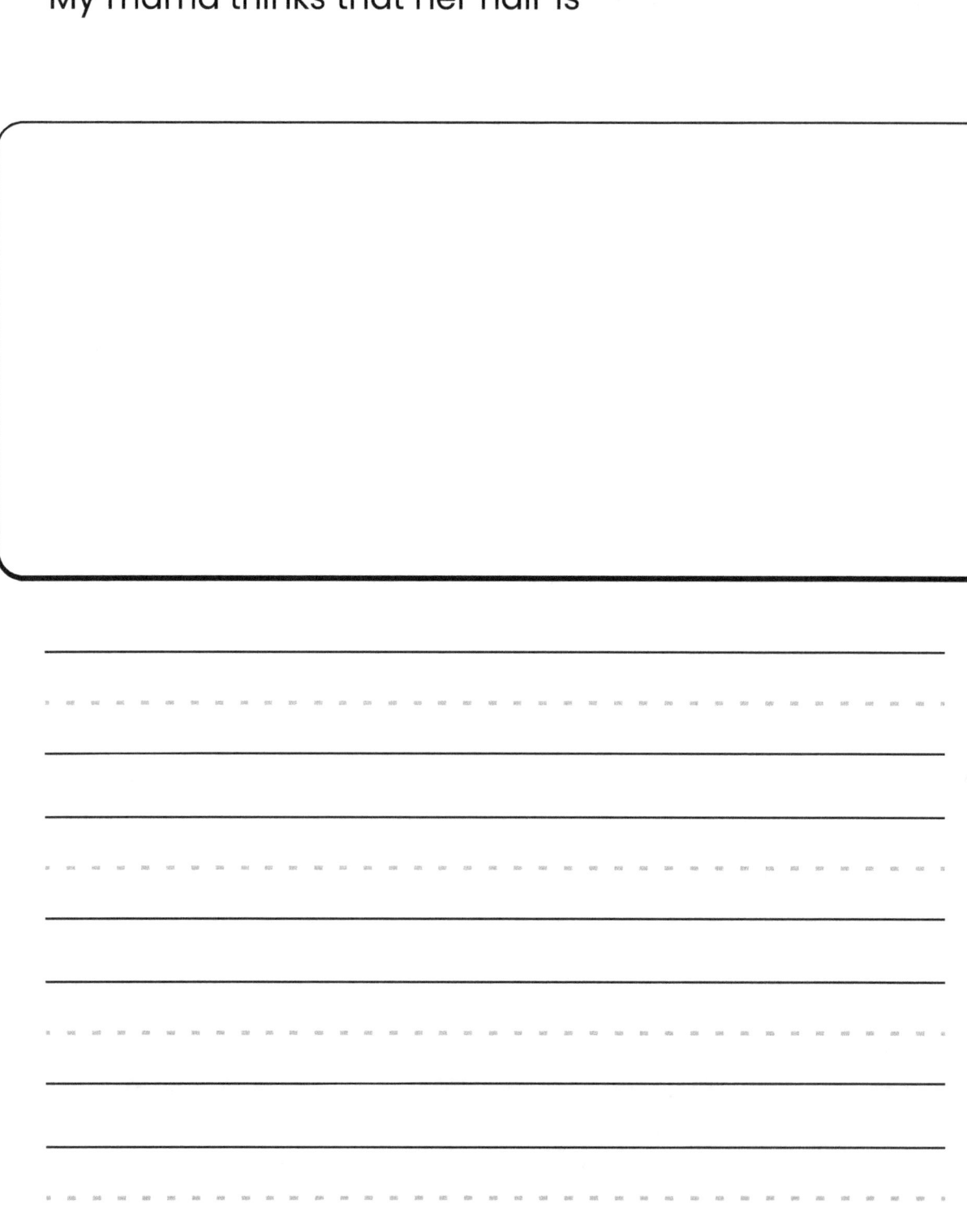

My mama thinks that my hair is

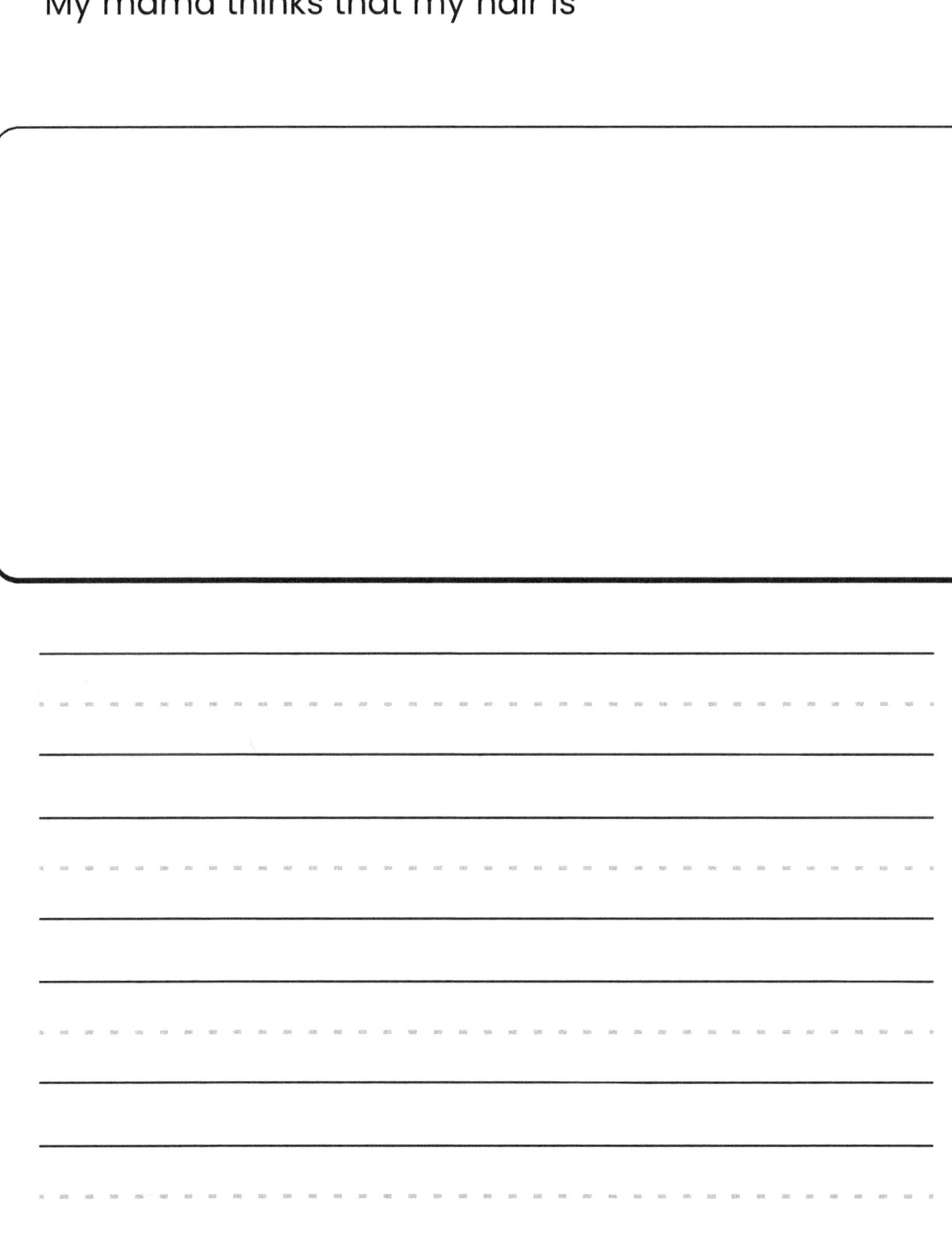

I think that my hair is